SMOOTHIE COOKBOOK FOR DIABETICS

Delicious smoothie recipes for diabetics

Table Of Contents

Table Of Contents	1
Terms Of Use Agreement	4
Disclaimer	5
Bunny Apple Smoothie	7
Dios Strawberry Breakfast	8
Caribbean Dream	9
Berries Full Of Protein	10
Vanilla and Peach Smoothie	11
Spinach, Orange & Kale Smoothie	12
Berries and Spinach Blaster	13
Banana Smoothie	14
Avocado and Banana Smoothie	15
Jamaican Fruit Smoothie	16
Refreshing Blast	17
Vanilla Smoothie	18
Diabetics Pina Colada	19
Spinach and Apple Freeze	20
Caramel and Peanut Smoothie	21

Strawberry Yogurt Smoothie	22
Almond and Honey Smoothie	23
Green Smoothie	24
Hel's Kitchen Smoothie	25
Morning Coffee Smoothie	26
Tofu, Strawberry, & Flax Seed Smoothie	27
Green Veggie Smoothie	28
Frozen Apple Smoothie	29
Hot Berry Smoothie	30
Cinnamon Green Smoothie	31
Green Banana Smoothie	32
Sweet Potato and Apple Smoothie	33
Pineapple and Kale Smoothie	34
Greek Smoothie	35
Coconut Green Smoothie	36
Orange and Fruit Smoothie	37
Vanilla Green Ice	38
Spinach and Lime Smoothie	39
Mango and Banana Smoothie	40
Grandma's Green Smoothie	41

Pomegranate and Berries Smoothie 42

Terms Of Use Agreement

Copyright 2014

All Rights Reserved

The author hereby asserts his/her right to be identified as the author of this work in accordance with sections 77 to 78 of the copyright, design and patents act 1988 as well as all other applicable international, federal, state and local laws.

Without limiting the rights under copyright reserved above, no part of this book may be reproduced, stored in or introduced into retrieval system, or transmitted, in any form or by any electronic or mechanical means, without the prior written permission of the copyright owner of this book, except by a reviewer who may quote brief passages.

There are no resale rights included. Anyone re - selling, or using this material in any way other than what is outlined within this book will be prosecuted to the full extend of the law.

Every effort had been made to fulfill requirements with regard to reproducing copyrighted material. The author and the publisher will be glad to certify any omissions at the earliest opportunity.

Disclaimer

The author and the publisher have used their best efforts in preparing this book. The author and the publisher make no representation or warranties with respect to the accuracy, fitness, applicability, or completeness of the contents of this work and specifically disclaim all warranties, including without limitation warranties of fitness for a particular purpose. This work is sold with the understanding that he author and the publisher is not engaged in rendering legal, or any other professional services.

The information contained in this book is strictly for educational purposes. Therefore, if you wish to apply ideas contained within this book, you are taking full responsibility for your actions. The author and the publisher disclaim any warranties (express or implied), merchantability, or fitness for any particular purpose. The Author and The publisher shall in no event be held responsible / liable to any party for any indirect, direct, special, punitive, incidental, or other consequential damages arising directly or indirectly from any use of this material, which is provided 'as is', and without warranties.

The author and the publisher do not warrant the performance, applicability, or effectiveness of any websites and other medias listed or linked to in this publication. All links are for informative purposes only and are not warranted for contents, accuracy, or any other implied or explicit purpose.

Bunny Apple Smoothie

Ingredients:

- 1 apple
- 1 banana
- 1 carrot
- 1 teaspoon of cinnamon powder
- 1 celery stick
- 1 sweet potato
- 1 lemon with skin
- 1/2 teaspoon of cayenne pepper
- 1 cup of fresh water.

Preparation:

- Blend all ingredients together until smooth.
- Enjoy!

Dios Strawberry Breakfast

Ingredients:

- 5 medium strawberries
- 1/2 cup low fat Greek-style yogurt
- 1 cup unsweetened soy milk
- 6 ice cubes

Preparation:

- Blend all ingredients together until smooth.
- Pour into a glass and garnish with a strawberry.
- Enjoy!

Caribbean Dream

Ingredients:

- 1 cup frozen blueberries
- 1 cup frozen raspberries
- 1 cup frozen blackberries
- 3 kale leaves
- small handful frozen mango chunks
- 2 cups unsweetened, pure coconut water
- 2 TBS flax meal

Preparation:

- Blend all ingredients together until smooth.
- Pour into glass and garnish with fresh berries.
- Enjoy!

Berries Full Of Protein

Ingredients:

- ¾ cup unsweetened almond milk
- ½ cup organic, wild blueberries, frozen
- 1/3 cup organic strawberries, frozen
- ½ avocado
- 1 handful organic spinach
- 1 tsp. organic flaxseed
- 1 scoop Vega Sports Protein
- 100g berry yogurt
- 1 tbsp. chia seeds
- 1 scoop greens superfood
- 4 ice cubes

Methods:

- Blend all ingredients together until smooth.
- Enjoy!

Vanilla and Peach Smoothie

Ingredients:

- 1 fresh peach, peeled, pitted, and chopped
- ½ cup skim milk
- 1 cup ice cubes
- 1 4-ounce carton non-fat vanilla yogurt
- ground cinnamon

Preparation:

- Blend all ingredients together until smooth.
- Pour into glass and sprinkle with cinnamon.
- Enjoy!

Spinach, Orange & Kale Smoothie

Ingredients:

- 1 small orange, peeled
- 2 big handfuls of spinach
- 1 large kale
- 1/2 cup frozen mixed berries
- 1 serving vegan protein powder
- 1 teaspoon goji berries, soaked for 10 minutes
- 1 teaspoon chia seeds
- 1 cup unsweetened organic coconut milk

Preparation:

- Blend all ingredients together until smooth.
- Use water to adjust consistency
- Enjoy!

Berries and Spinach Blaster

Preparation:

- 2 cups spinach
- 1/2 cup strawberries
- 1/2 cup blueberries
- 1 scoop of sugar free chocolate protein powder
- 1 tablespoon of ground flax seed
- 1/4 cup soaked chia seed
- 1 teaspoon of ground cinnamon
- A small handful of raw pumpkin seeds

Ingredients:

- Blend all ingredients together until smooth.
- Enjoy!

Banana Smoothie

Ingredients:

- 2 ounces of spinach
- 2 ounces of kale
- 1 ounce of hemp seeds
- 1.5 - 2 cups of water

Preparation:

- Blend all ingredients together until smooth.
- Enjoy!

Avocado and Banana Smoothie

Ingredients:

- 8 oz unsweetened almond milk
- 2-3 cups of spinach
- 1 medium banana, peeled
- 1/2 small avocado

Preparation:

- Blend all ingredients together until smooth.
- Enjoy!

Jamaican Fruit Smoothie

Ingredients:

- 1 cucumber
- 1 stalk of celery
- cup Kale
- 2 cups frozen fruit chunks of your choice
- 1 frozen banana, peeled
- 1/2 small avocado
- 1 lemon, peeled
- 16 ounces water

Preparation:

- Blend all ingredients together until smooth.
- Enjoy!

Refreshing Blast

Ingredients:

- Ice water
- Handful dandelion greens
- Handful chickweed
- Several sprigs of mint
- Several sprigs of parsley
- 3 small leaves spinach
- Half of avocado
- 2 teaspoons of chia seeds
- ½ cup of plain yogurt
- Frozen berries

Preparation:

- Blend all ingredients together until smooth.
- Enjoy!

Vanilla Smoothie

Ingredients:

- 1 cup almond milk, unsweetened
- ½ cup Hood Calorie Countdown Dairy Beverage
- 2 packets Splenda
- ½ small banana
- 2 tablespoons DaVinci Strawberry Sugar Free Syrup
- 1 teaspoon Jello Sugar-free Vanilla Pudding Singles powder
- 1 tablespoon PaleoFiber powder
- 1 scoop of vanilla protein powder

Preparation:

- Blend all ingredients together until smooth.
- Enjoy!

Diabetics Pina Colada

Ingredients:

- 1 cup light plain yogurt
- 1 cup fresh or canned pineapple
- 1 tsp. coconut flavor
- 1 cup crushed ice

Preparation:

- Blend all ingredients together until smooth.
- Enjoy!

Spinach and Apple Freeze

Ingredients:

- 1 cup almond milk
- 2 large handfuls of fresh spinach
- 1-2 scoops of protein powder
- 1 banana, preferably frozen
- 1 Tbsp. frozen apple juice concentrate
- 6-8 ice cubes

Preparation:

- Blend all ingredients together until smooth.
- Enjoy!

Caramel and Peanut Smoothie

Ingredients:

- 1 cup almond milk, unsweetened
- ½ cup of skim milk
- 2 packets Splenda
- 1 tablespoon unsweetened cocoa powder
- 1 tablespoon DaVinci Caramel Sugar Free Syrup
- 1 tablespoon creamy peanut butter
- 1 tablespoon ground flaxseed meal
- ¾ scoop vanilla protein powder

Preparation:

- Blend all ingredients together until smooth.
- Enjoy!

Strawberry Yogurt Smoothie

Ingredients:

- 1 cup fresh or frozen whole strawberries
- 1 banana
- 1 cup light and sugar-free strawberry yogurt
- 1 cup crushed ice

Preparation:

- Blend all ingredients together until smooth.
- Enjoy!

Almond and Honey Smoothie

Ingredients:

- 1-1/2 cups fresh blueberries
- 1/2 cup plain fat-free Greek yogurt
- 1/4 cup slivered almonds
- 2 tablespoons wheat germ
- 2 tablespoons unsweetened almond milk
- 2 teaspoons honey
- 1 cup ice cubes

Preparation:

- Blend all ingredients together until smooth.
- Enjoy!

Green Smoothie

Ingredients:

- 1 pkg. sugar substitute
- 2 tsps. Matcha green tea powder
- 1 cup skim milk
- 1 banana
- 3 tbsps. hot water
- 1 cup crushed ice
- 1 tsp. mint extract

Preparation:

- Blend all ingredients together until smooth.
- Enjoy!

Hel's Kitchen Smoothie

Ingredients:

- 1 & ½ cup of fresh raspberries
- 2 tablespoons skim milk
- 2 tablespoons natural smooth peanut butter
- 2 teaspoons honey
- 1 cup ice cubes

Preparation:

- Blend all ingredients together until smooth.
- Enjoy!

Morning Coffee Smoothie

Ingredients:

- 1/2 cup uncooked oats
- 1 frozen banana (small chunks)
- 1 tbsp. ground flaxseed
- 1 pkg. sugar substitute
- 1 1/2 cup skim milk
- 1 tsp. coffee flavor

Preparation:

- Blend all ingredients together until smooth.
- Enjoy!

Tofu, Strawberry, & Flax Seed Smoothie

Ingredients:

- 1-1/2 cups fresh strawberries
- 1/2 medium banana, sliced
- 1/2 cup soft tofu
- 2 tablespoons of ground flax seeds
- 2 tablespoons of skim milk
- 2 teaspoons of honey
- 1 cup of ice cubes

Preparation:

- Blend all ingredients together until smooth.
- Enjoy!

Green Veggie Smoothie

Ingredients:

- 1 cup almond milk, unsweetened
- 1/4 red bell pepper, sliced
- 1/4 teaspoon turmeric
- 1/2 banana
- 1/2 tablespoon coconut oil
- 4 strawberries, chopped
- shake cinnamon

Preparation:

- Blend all ingredients together until smooth.
- Enjoy!

Frozen Apple Smoothie

Ingredients:

- 1 small apple, cored and chopped
- 2 cups of baby spinach
- 1/2 cup plain fat-free Greek yogurt
- 1/3 cup unsweetened apple juice
- 2 tablespoons ground flax seeds
- 1 teaspoon maple syrup
- 1 cup ice cubes

Preparation:

- Blend all ingredients together until smooth.
- Enjoy!

Hot Berry Smoothie

Ingredients:

- 1 ½ cup of fresh raspberries
- 1/2 cup of fat-free cottage cheese
- 2 pitted dates
- 2 tablespoons of rolled oats
- 1 teaspoon honey
- Pinch of ground cinnamon
- 1 cup ice cubes

Preparation:

- Blend all ingredients together until smooth.
- Enjoy!

Cinnamon Green Smoothie

Ingredients:

- 6 ounces of unsweetened almond milk
- Handful of spinach
- 3 slices of cucumber
- 3 tablespoon of organic rolled oats
- 1 tablespoon of flaxseed
- 1/2 stalk of celery
- 1 teaspoon of organic cinnamon
- 2 frozen strawberries
- 1/2 cup of blueberries
- 1 tablespoon of raw cacao

Preparation:

- Blend all ingredients together until smooth.
- Enjoy!

Green Banana Smoothie

Ingredients:

- 1 head baby bok choy
- 1 cup kale
- 1 red plum, pitted
- 1 medium banana, peeled
- 1/4 avocado

Preparation:

- Blend all ingredients together until smooth.
- Enjoy!

Sweet Potato and Apple Smoothie

Ingredients:

- 1 sweet potato
- 1 banana
- 1 lemon with skin
- 1 carrot
- 1 apple
- 1 celery stick
- 1 teaspoon of cinnamon powder
- 1/2 teaspoon of cayenne pepper
- 1 cup of fresh water.

Preparation:

- Blend all ingredients together until smooth.
- Enjoy!

Pineapple and Kale Smoothie

Ingredients:

- 1 and 1/2 cups kale
- 1/2 cup parsley
- 2 cups fresh pineapple
- 1 cups whole strawberries
- 1 medium banana, peeled
- 1 Tbsp Hemp seeds

Preparation:

- Blend all ingredients together until smooth.
- Enjoy!

Greek Smoothie

Ingredients:

- 1 cup of unsweetened soymilk
- 5 medium fresh or frozen strawberries
- ½ cup of low-fat Greek yogurt
- some ice cubes

Preparation:

- Blend all ingredients together until smooth.
- Enjoy!

Coconut Green Smoothie

Ingredients:

- 1 cup coconut milk
- 3 tablespoons cacao powder
- ½ of avocado
- 2 cups of ice

Preparation:

- Blend all ingredients together until smooth.
- Enjoy!

Orange and Fruit Smoothie

Ingredients:

- 16 oz Plain Yogurt
- 12 oz Mixed Berries
- 1/4 tsp Vanilla Extract
- 1/2 cup Ice
- 1/2 cup Orange Juice
- 1/4 cup Strawberries
- 1 tbsp Granular

Preparation:

- Blend together yogurt, berries, sugar substitute, and vanilla.
- Add juice and the ice cubes.
- Blend together until smooth.
- Enjoy!

Vanilla Green Ice

Ingredients:

- 1 cup almond milk
- 7 drops stevia
- 2 cups spinach
- 1 and 1/2 teaspoons of vanilla extract
- 2 cups of ice

Preparation:

- Blend all ingredients together until smooth.
- Enjoy!

Spinach and Lime Smoothie

Ingredients:

- juice of 4 limes
- zest of 2 limes
- 2 cups of spinach leaves
- some ice cubes
- 1 tbsp of sunflower butter

Preparation:

- Blend all ingredients together until smooth.
- Enjoy!

Mango and Banana Smoothie

Ingredients:

- 1 cup of tinned mango
- 1 tbsp honey
- 1 banana
- 1 reduced fat greek-style yogurt
- 2 tsp wheat germ

Preparation:

- Blend all ingredients together until smooth.
- Enjoy!

Grandma's Green Smoothie

Ingredients:

- Handful of spinach
- 3 slices of cucumber
- 1/2 stalk of celery
- 1 teaspoon of organic cinnamon
- 2 frozen strawberries
- 1 tablespoon of flaxseed
- 1/2 cup of blueberries
- 3 tablespoon of organic rolled oats
- 1 tablespoon of raw cacao
- 6 ounces of unsweetened almond milk

Preparation:

- Blend all ingredients together until smooth.
- Enjoy!

Pomegranate and Berries Smoothie

Ingredients:

- 1 cup Low Fat Greek Yogurt
- 1 cup Pomegranate Cranberry Juice
- 10 Blackberries
- 10 Raspberries
- 10 Strawberries, Sliced
- 1 Banana, Sliced & Peeled

Preparation:

- Blend all ingredients together until smooth.
- Enjoy!

Printed in the USA
CPSIA information can be obtained
at www.ICGtesting.com
LVHW012036140524
780250LV00002B/455